Moses BADIANJILE

Management of vasoocclusive crises in sickle cell disease patients

Moses BADIANJILE

Management of vasoocclusive crises in sickle cell disease patients

Management of vaso occlusive seizures in sickle cell children aged 6 months to 17 years CMMASS/DRC cases

ScienciaScripts

Imprint

Cover image: www.ingimage.com

This book is a translation from the original published under ISBN 978-613-8-42922-7.

Publisher:
Sciencia Scripts
is a trademark of
Dodo Books Indian Ocean Ltd. and OmniScriptum S.R.L publishing group

120 High Road, East Finchley, London, N2 9ED, United Kingdom
Str. Armeneasca 28/1, office 1, Chisinau MD-2012, Republic of Moldova, Europe
Managing Directors: Ieva Konstantinova, Victoria Ursu
info@omniscriptum.com

Printed at: see last page
ISBN: 978-620-8-62726-3

DEDICATION

TO MY GOD

Master of times and circumstances, despite our weaknesses and conduct he has extended

his powerful hand on me and my supervisors to make this work a success.

TO MY MOTHER MUSELA TSHIBANGU MADO

An attentive, simple, courageous and pious mother, you taught me good manners and the advantages of a job well done. The great love of a job well done that you instilled in me helped me a great deal in carrying out this work.

IN MEMORY OF MY FATHER BADIANJILE KENA CELESTIN

You were torn from the affection of us all, and your death was a great loss to me. You only get a father once in your life, and I've come to understand that.

I wish you could have been with us today to share this long-awaited joy, but GOD decided otherwise.

TO MY MENTOR AND CO-DIRECTOR JEPHTE BAMBI

A supervisor who is available and understanding, despite his multiple occupations and the other students under his supervision, he knows how to give time to everyone. The guidelines they give me for my work have always worked.

ACKNOWLEDGEMENTS

I thank GOD for allowing us to reach the end of our work.

I would like to thank all the people who have helped me any way, both during my studies and during this work:

TO THE PASTORAL COUPLE TUJIBIKILE TSHIBANGU

Your support at every level, your encouragement and your affection have failed me.

TO MY LITTLE SISTER KENA KENA ESPERANCE AND HER HUSBAND KONGOLO SAMY

I have never missed your support, especially your financial support. Rest assured of my deep love.

A MA TANTINE BAMUBILE TSHIBANGU Godée

I have never missed your support, especially your financial support. Rest assured of my deep love.

TO ALL MY BROTHERS AND SISTERS ON MY MOTHER AND FATHER'S SIDE

For your encouragement and wishes for success. TO MY PROFESSOR DIRECTOR Dr. BODI
A great man in the world of science, a man who has trained many elders but who accepted that I should also be among his disciples, I'm really delighted about that.

TSHIBANGU AND KENA FAMILIES

I 't mention any names for fear of forgetting some. Thank you for all your support.

CONTENTS

SUMMARY

This was a documentary and retrospective study over 12 months, carried out in a paediatric setting in Kinshasa. The general objective was to evaluate the method of pain treatment by analgesic increments recommended by the World Health Organization (WHO) for sickle cell pain.

The study involved 220 sickle cell patients of both sexes, aged between 6 months and 17 years, who were experiencing a painful crisis. The average duration of treatment was 5 days, depending on the severity of the painful symptoms.

Pain intensity was assessed using the EVA (visual analogue scale) and DEGR (pain enfant Goustave Roussy) scales.

The effectiveness of analgesic treatment was systematically assessed at the 2nd hour. The 6-10 age was the most affected (40%). In 52.27% of cases, pain was relieved by a level I analgesic (Paracetamol) and 47.73% by a level II analgesic (Temgesic).

In 50% of our patients, the pain subsided in more than 12 hours, with an average of 9 hours, compared with only 31.8% who subsided in less than 12 hours.

The less intense the pain, the shorter the sedation period.

INTRODUCTION

1 PROBLEM STATEMENT :

Sickle cell anaemia comes from two Greek words "DREPANON" which means It is also called "FAUCILLE" and "CYTOS" which means "CELLULE"(1). "SS anaemia", referring to the type of haemoglobin found in the blood(2). Or This is called "sickle cell anaemia" because of the sickle-shaped appearance of the affected red blood cell(1). This is an inherited disorder characterised by a structural anomaly in haemoglobin responsible for a polymerisation process in a deoxygenation situation *1, 2+.It is real pain disease and the cause of repeated, sometimes unbearable, painful attacks, dreaded by parents and often inadequately treated *3+. A complex disease, its course is still difficult to predict despite better knowledge of the risks and increasingly organised prevention. In addition to the genetic polymorphism, the clinical polymorphism of this disease calls on multiple clinical and biological skills, which may justify treating these patients in specialised centres *4+. Sickle cell anaemia affects more than 100 million people worldwide(6), and is the haemoglobinopathy most commonly found in blacks(4,5), accounting for 9% of black Americans and 12% of blacks in the West Indies. It is also found in certain Arab and European countries, with prevalence in Europe estimated at around 1/850 *6,7) In France, the number children suffering from the disease thought to be around 3,000, in Italy 2,850 and in Greece 2,500 *3, 4+.In Africa, it is the most common genetic disease and therefore a real public health problem. Two hundred thousand children with sickle cell disease are born every year, and half of them die before the age of 5(7). In North Africa, around 5% of the population has sickle cell disease. In West Africa, the incidence is as high as 20%(9). In Mali, the prevalence of sickle cell disease is estimated at 12% on average, with the major form accounting for 1 to 3% [8]. In Central Africa, particularly the DRC, Congo Brazzaville and Nigeria, 40% of the population suffer from this haemoglobinopathy. Sickle cell disease a genetic disorder with an estimated prevalence of 2% in the general population in the Democratic Republic of Congo (DRC)(29). In Africa, the high morbidity and mortality associated with this disease is due to precarious socio-economic conditions, a lack of organisation and equipment in health facilities, and a shortage of qualified medical staff [5]. One of the WHO's priorities is the fight against pain. With this in mind, at a WHO conference in Milan in 1982, the method treating pain by stages of analgesics was developed, and has since become a WHO recommendation for pain control worldwide [6].

2. JUSTIFICATION FOR STUDY

In the DRC, as in several other countries, the painful crisis is the leading cause of admission of sickle cell patients to hospital and is the very symbol of violent pain in paediatrics. It responsible for frequent and sometimes prolonged hospitalisation, as well as school absenteeism*6,7+.

3. PURPOSE OF THE STUDY :

In view of the above, we thought it would be useful to initiate this study on vaso-occlusive crises in order to help improve the management of this pain in children with sickle cell disease in our community.

4. OBJECTIVES

4.1. GENERAL OBJECTIVE :

To evaluate the management of vaso-occlusive crises in children with sickle cell disease admitted to the SS Mixed Medicine and Anaemia Centre.

4.2. SPECIFIC OBJECTIVES :

➢ Determine the frequency of attacks vaso-occlusive attacks at the sickle-cell anaemia children admitted to the SS.
➢ Describe the socio-demographic characteristics of these sickle cell patients.
➢ Describe their clinical picture admission.
➢ Specify the pain relief treatment in place.
➢ Determine their clinical course.

GENERAL

II.1. GENERAL INFORMATION ON SICKLE CELL DISEASE :

II.1.1. Definition: *10+

Sickle cell anaemia is a genetic disease defined by the presence of abnormal haemoglobin (HbS) in the red blood cells. It is a qualitative haemoglobinopathy mainly of the black race, the pathogenesis of which involves a point mutation at codon number 6 of the globin beta chain of the hydrophilic glutamate residue of adult haemoglobin A by a hydrophobic valine residue. This reduces the solubility of haemoglobin, which tends to precipitate.

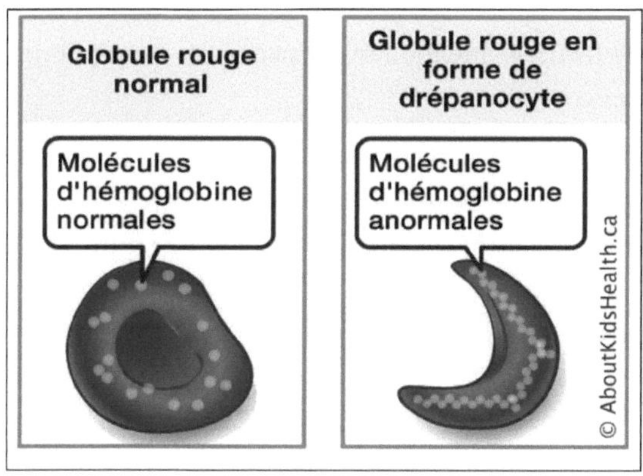

Normal red blood cells are biconcave, circular and pass easily through the blood capillaries thanks to shape and flexibility; healthy red blood cells are able to change shape in order to pass through the vessels. When they no longer have the right shape and resemble a sickle, their flexibility and ability to change shape in the blood vessels are no longer possible. Abnormal red blood cells resemble a sickle, a curved farming tool, like a semicircular blade. They are often described as having a crescent moon shape, and it is the change in the shape of the red blood cells that ultimately leads to the many medical conditions.

II.1.2. History: [6, 8, 9, 10,11]

Known for a very long time in the African medical tradition, sickle cell anaemia was only studied in the twentieth century, initially in black Americans. In 1910 HERRICK defined the disease as a new clinical entity, described the sickle-shaped appearance of the red blood cells and explained the anaemia by their hyperhaemolysis.

In 1917 EMMEL discovered that the red blood cells of sickle cell patients kept for a certain period of time protected from the air became sickle cell (principle of the EMMEL test), a phenomenon not observed in normal subjects.

In 1949 Pauling demonstrated the abnormal nature of haemoglobin using electrophoresis, thus describing the first molecular disease. In the 1950s, DIGGS contributed to the precise clinical description of the various manifestations of the disease.

In 1957 INGRAM showed that haemoglobin S differed from adult haemoglobin A (HbA) by only one amino acid, namely the sixth amino acid from the hydrophilic N-terminus of its beta chain.

In 1966 ROBINSON drew attention to the particular susceptibility of these subjects to pneumococcus.

In 1969 PEARSON individualised the concept functional asplenia. And from 1972 onwards, prenatal diagnosis of the disease was envisaged by KAN and VALENTI, and by SOUTHERM in 1978 through the study of DNA.

II.1.3. REMINDER OF HAEMOGLOBINOGENESIS:(27)

Haemoglobin, the coloured pigment that gives red blood cells their red colour, accounts for 95% of intracellular proteins. The physiological role of haemoglobin is primarily to transport oxygen from the lungs to the tissues, but it also facilitates the elimination of carbon dioxide.

- **Structure haemoglobin :**

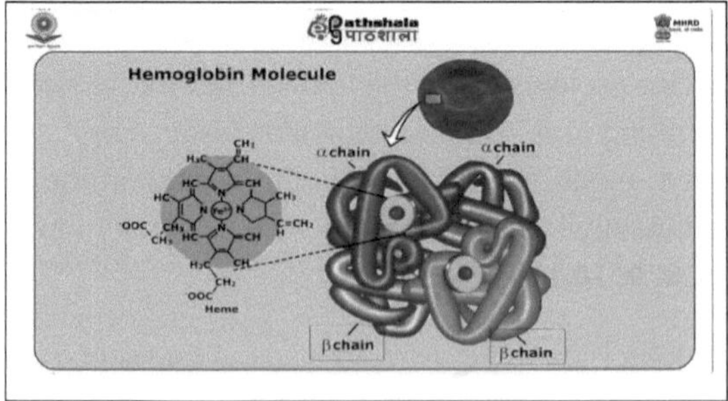

It's a structure cyclic organic complex comprising a prosthetic group, heme, and a protein part, globin.

Heme

It is formed by protoporphyrin IX, to which an iron atom is bound in the ferrous state. Protoporphyrin is made up of 4 pyrrole rings linked by methenyl bridges. The iron in the heme binds to the four nitrogen atoms at the centre of the protoporphyrin nucleus forms two other coordinating bonds on side of the heme plane. Oxygen can only bind to the heme if it is in the ferrous state. A heme is linked to a globin chain and forms a subunit. The four sub-units fit together to form a tetrahedron: the haemoglobin molecule.

Globin chains

There are two types of globin chain family: α-family chains and β-family chains. It is the nature of the chains that defines haemoglobin. In fact, there is always a pairing of two α-type chains with two β-type chains. Haemoglobin production in humans is characterised by two major changes in the composition of haemoglobin.

- During embryonic life, there are two types of α chain: The ζ chain, which appears first, and then the α chain. Similarly, there are two types of β family chains: the ε chain specific to this period and the γ (or foetal) chain. Consequently, in the embryo, there are 3 types of haemoglobin: Gower 1 (ζ2 ε2), Gower 2 (α2) and Portland (ζ 22).
- Fetal haemoglobin (HbF) structure (α2 γ2) is detectable from the fifth week of intrauterine life. Its synthesis reaches a rate of 90% between the 8th and 10th week (more or less constant until birth). The transition from foetal haemoglobin to adult haemoglobin occurs during the perinatal period, and ends at the end of the first year of life.
- Normal haemoglobin in adults is made up mainly of HbA (α2 β2) for around 97%, a small fraction of HbA2 (α2 δ2) for 2 to 3% and traces of HbF (α2 γ2), less than 1%.

- Haemoglobin function

Haemoglobin transports molecular oxygen (O2) from the lungs to the tissues and carbon dioxide (CO2) from the tissues to the lungs. Its affinity for O2 varies according to its partial pressure (PO2). This affinity, modulated by the heme-heme interactions of the tetrahedral structure, is mediocre at low PO2, which allows O2 to be delivered to the tissues. It increases considerably at high PO2, and the haemoglobin dissociation curve has a characteristic sigmoidal shape. 2,3-Diphosphoglycerate (2,3 DPG), formed during anaerobic glycolysis, binds to the central cavity of deoxygenated Haemoglobin as the α1-β2 and α2- β1 bonds loosen. This binding leads to a drop in the affinity of haemoglobin for O2. Normally, the P50 (PO2 at which haemoglobin is 50% saturated) is 26 mm Hg. In vivo, the arterial O2 content is 95mmHg with 95% saturation, while venous blood has a partial pressure of 40mmHg and 70% saturation.

II.1.4. GENETICS :

II.1.4.1. Genetic characterisation :

Sickle cell disease is inherited in the autosomal Co dominant mode. For the clinician, it appears to be recessive because only homozygotes are seriously ill; for the biochemist, it is dominant because haemoglobin S is present in both heterozygotes and homozygotes at obviously different levels *6+. It occurs in a child with an alteration (mutation) in both copies of the gene involved in haemoglobin production [6,12].

One of these copies is inherited from the father and the other from the mother; more often than not, the parents do not themselves have sickle cell disease, but one of the copies of the gene is altered in both of them. A genomic study can then be envisaged, the PCR method, which is a DNA amplification technique used to identify a haemoglobinopathy *6; 12].

II.1.4.2. Genetic prognostic factors or haplotypes [6,9].

Haplo-types are the combination of several restriction sites (i.e. specific base sequences) on the βs gene. Five of them, namely the Bantu, Beninese, Cameroonian, Arab-Indian and Senegalese haplotypes, are thought to be prognostic determinants of sickle cell disease because of their linkage disequilibrium with the βs mutation. They are thought to reduce the overall severity of the disease.

II.1.5. Epidemiology :

The ethnic and geographical distribution of sickle cell disease is remarkable. Black Africans in the sickle belt, which stretches from the 15th parallel of north latitude to the 20th parallel of south latitude, are the most affected. It is sometimes seen in non-melanoderma subjects in the Middle East, Saudi Arabia,

Greece and North Africa, where it is often associated with other haemoglobinopathies such as thalassaemia and haemoglobin C *6+. As a result of the movement of the African population towards Western Europe, sickle cell disease is now present in France, England, Portugal, Belgium, the Netherlands and Germany*10+. The coincidence between sickle cell endemic areas and malaria infestation areas has led to the hypothesis that heterozygous AS sickle cell patients have a selective advantage over normal AA individuals with regard to malaria *6+.

II.1.6. PATHOPHYSIOLOGY :

➢ **Falciformation :**

Oxygenated haemoglobin S is as soluble as adult Hb A; but it is less stable and polymerises when deoxygenated: formation of crystals, *3+ gelation. In heterozygous sickle cell patients, the erythrocyte concentration of HbS is too low for falciformation to occur. On the other hand, in SS subjects, falciformation occurs easily in capillaries favoured by acidosis, dehydration, fever, hypoxia, intense effort or stress*3,6+. Numerous studies have all concluded that there is a highly variable delay from one red blood cell to another in the phenomenon of polymerisation and then falciformation when they are subjected to low Po2. The study was repeated in concentrated Hb solution and it was shown that the main factor influencing polymerisation time was Hb concentration. This highlighted the importance of the Hb concentration of red blood cells in the development of a deformability disorder likely to lead to defective perfusion of micro-vessels. This observation has been made clinically useful through considerations on the importance of good cellular hydration *13].

➢ **Thrombosis and haemolysis :**

This is explained by the presence of rigid sickle cells, which increase the viscosity of the blood and therefore the transit time in the capillaries, where they clump together, leading to occlusion of the microcirculation and infarctions*10+. In addition, sickle cells are fragile and are destroyed prematurely by the reticuloendothelial system. It should be noted that the lifespan of a sickle cell erythrocyte is 10 to 12 days, compared with 120 days for a normal *6+ erythrocyte. The frequency of infections in sickle cell disease can be explained by the existence of visceral infarcts where bacteria multiply. Immune defences as such appear to be little affected *10+.

II.1.7. . Semiology: [11]

In the normal state and in the absence of complications, the disease results in chronic haemolytic anaemia, which is generally well tolerated. Pallor is often clearly visible in the mucous membranes. Anemia is fairly well tolerated in everyday life, and patients are more or less normally active. However, the situation deteriorates rapidly during prolonged exertion, particularly in sports, or when there is a sudden change in temperature. Conjunctival jaundice is common, clearly due to hyperhaemolysis. Splenomegaly appears early in the course of the disease, at around 6 months. It is firm and remains palpable until 6-8 years of age, at which time it usually begins to involute and is no longer clinically noticeable by 8-10 years of age. In sickle cell disease, there is therefore a genuine auto-splenectomy which can be linked to the progressive involution of the organ and its fibrosis, sometimes with calcifications due to multiple and repeated micro-infarctions.

The spleen can play an unfavourable role in the course of the disease in 3 ways:

- by the loss of its functional value during childhood which can lead to infections;

- by slowing intra-splenic circulation promoting haemolysis;

- lastly, it may increase in volume progressively or abruptly and sequester a large proportion of the blood mass; this is therefore a crisis of splenic sequestration, the seriousness of which must be emphasised. The liver may be normal, but is often only moderately enlarged, palpable to within a few centimetres of the costal crest; a larger enlargement may occur during the course of the disease, but this should be investigated as a complication.

II.1.8.1. Vaso-occlusive crisis: (see point 1.2.)

II.1.8.2. Anemia :

In general, the basal Hb level of sickle cell patients is stable at between 6.5 and 9g/dl. This chronic anaemia is well tolerated *4+. Against this background of chronic haemolysis, the evolution of major sickle cell syndromes may be punctuated by episodes of acute anaemia, the main mechanisms of which are *5+ :

• Hyperhaemolytic crisis: Episodes of haemolytic crisis can occur at any age *5+. They are often associated with an infectious process, in particular malaria in our context, or a G6PD deficiency *5,6+. Treatment consists a simple transfusion of packed red blood cells or, failing that, whole blood *5+.

• Crises of splenic sequestration: These are common in infants and small children *5+. The onset is abrupt and marked by sudden onset of anaemiajaundice, hypovolaemic collapse splenomegaly with sequestration of most of the red blood cells *6+.

The course of the disease is rapidly fatal, requiring early and appropriate management based on emergency blood transfusion*5,6+.

Death occurs in the absence of transfusion; if there is survival, recurrences are frequent and may lead to splenectomy being considered, or a transfusion programme being initiated [5,6].

Indeed, in the absence of neonatal screening and systematic Hb electrophoresis in newborns of mothers with a positive EMMEL test, it is likely that infants with this type of complication died before sickle cell disease *5+ was diagnosed.

• Acute transient erythroblastopenia: This can occur at any age and usually follows a nasopharyngeal infection; parvovirus B19 is the classic cause*5,6+. It is diagnosed by a rapid worsening of the anaemia, which is regenerative with no increase in jaundice or spleen volume, associated with little or no reticulocytosis *5+. Recovery is usually spontaneous, but a blood transfusion is often necessary until erythropoiesis is restored *5,6+.

Its indication takes into account the fall in baseline Hb level and the clinical tolerance of the anaemia *5+.

II.1.8.3. **Infectious complications :**

They are extremely common and remain the main cause of morbidity and mortality in children with sickle cell disease, particularly in childhood [6,14].

They punctuate the course of a sickle-cell anaemic child's life, often putting him or her at risk. In infants, even a trivial viral infection can suddenly trigger acute or sub-acute splenic sequestration *6+. They are also responsible for vaso-occlusive crises through fever, hypoxia and dehydration, which are all factors in sickle cell disease *8+. Hence the vicious circle between infection and sickle cell disease. The most common infections are pneumonia, meningitis and septicaemia, osteomyelitis and, to a lesser extent, urinary tract and intestinal infections. The germs involved are varied, but some are clearly dominant: pneumococcus, salmonella, but also haemophilus influenzae b and mycoplasma [11]. Post-transfusion viral infections such as HIV and hepatitis B and C *5+ may also be observed.

II.1.8. .4. Serious vaso-occlusive accidents :

The most typical and frequent manifestations major sickle cell syndromes are : *5+

II.1.8.4.1. Neurological manifestations

These are dominated by damage to the CNS, particularly strokes, and account for a significant proportion of general mortality linked to sickle cell disease. They tend to recur and often lead to persistent and disabling neurological sequelae *8+. Strokes can occur at any age, although they are slightly more common in younger people. Two types of anatomical lesions may be observed.

• Cerebral infarctions: These are caused by partial or complete obstruction of the large intracranial vessels. The clinical symptomatology, which is usually brutal, is marked by headaches, convulsions, sometimes behavioural problems, followed by the appearance of hemiplegia and possibly aphasia within a few hours or days. In some cases coma may occur, but this is uncommon *8+.

• Intracranial haemorrhage: This is rare and exceptional in children with sickle cell disease. They generally occur between the ages of 14 and 36, with an average age of 25, and usually have a sudden onset with coma and hemiplegia preceded by a short period of often violent headaches *8+. From a therapeutic point of view, the introduction of a lifelong transfusion programme is the only method of preventing recurrences, the effectiveness of which is unanimously recognised *5+.

II.1.8.4.2. Acute chest syndrome (ACS): (see point 1.2.) II.1.8.4.3. Priapism: (see point 1.2.)

II.1.8.5. Bone complications: Following a CVO, two complications may be feared:

• Bone infarction: This is secondary to obliteration of a medium-calibre artery and sometimes occurs after the attack. A bone crisis lasts 3 to 5 days. Persistent bone pain, especially if accompanied by local inflammatory signs, is highly suggestive infarction. The most dangerous location is the head femoral bone, which is easily necrotic due to a significant reduction in its blood supply [4].

• Osteomyelitis: A haematogenous infection of the bone, it is mainly due to salmonella, against which sickle cell patients have poor defence *4,15+.

It often follows CVO and develops within a bone infarct. Diagnosis of these two types of bone damage is very difficult. As the treatment is very different, it is important to be able to use bone scintigraphy *4+.
1.8. Chronic complications: These appear in childhood and their frequency tends to increase with age. They are mainly linked to chronic haemolysis, ischaemia and anaemia*5+.

II.1.8.6. Biliary lithiasis

This is often asymptomatic and should be investigated by abdominal ultrasound at least once a year from the age of 5*5+.

Symptomatically, a sometimes painful hepatomegaly and pigmented biliary lithiasis are observed on abdominal ultrasound *6+. In terms of treatment, some authors advocate abstention and monitoring because stones are asymptomatic for a long time; others, on the contrary, recommend systematic cholecystectomy to avoid acute complications requiring emergency treatment with uncertain results [5].

II.1.8.7. Retinopathy

Asymptomatic for a long time, it should be systematically sought in sickle cell patients. It generally appears in adolescence and occurs earlier in SC patients than in SS patients *8+. Diagnosis is based on retinal angiography. Treatment of retinopathy consists of laser photo coagulation from the stage of capillary proliferation (stage III) to prevent vitreous haemorrhage (stage IV) and retinal detachment (stage V) *5+. However, given the rarity of visual deficits, the high cost of laser treatment and the risk of complications, this indication should be treated with caution.

II.1.8.8. Osteonecrosis

This is one of the most serious complications of sickle cell disease and forms part of the chronic complications of this disease. Aseptic epiphyseal osteonecrosis is common in sickle cell disease, mainly affecting the femoral head, but also the humeral head, femoral condyle, tibial plateau, talus and tarsal bones. Femoral head disease is the most serious in functional terms. Bone scans can provide an early indication of osteonecrosis of the femoral head *15+. The longer life expectancy of these patients, and sometimes the delay in diagnosis, means that relatively large numbers of degenerative osteoarthritic lesions appear in adulthood [15]. Treatment consists of simple off-loading and monitoring by the orthopaedic team with a view to possible surgical cure *5+.

II.1.8.9. Leg ulcer

This is favoured by a low baseline Hb and HbF level, which may explain its relative rarity in our patients. Treatment consists of protective dressings which allow healing, but recurrence may occur after one year in both cases *5+.

II.1.8.8. Cardiac damage

*16+ These are the consequences of chronic anaemia and repeated micro infarctions. Ischaemic complications are common in children with homozygous sickle cell disease, but the heart does not appear to be the target organ.

Early detection of myocardial ischaemia in these children could prevent cardiac complications. Specific treatment of sickle cell disease with hydroxyurea is discussed in the presence of clear abnormalities in myocardial perfusion.

II.1.8.9. Renal manifestations:[17]

• Decreased urine concentration: This is a constant feature in homozygous subjects and is rare in heterozygotes. It leads to polyuria of 2 to 3 litres/day. There is therefore a risk of dehydration, which is a factor in triggering sickle cell disease.

• Haematuria: this may be micro or macroscopic. It is common in sickle cell disease, especially in young people. - Urinary tract infections: The sickle cell patient's deficient immunity and hypovascularisation favour infections. The sickle cell patient's environment must be healthy because it can be a reservoir for germs.

• Other symptoms include acute or chronic renal failure and nephrotic syndrome.

II.1.9. Diagnosis of sickle cell disease :

It is essentially biological. It should be suspected in the presence of any clinical or biological anaemia, recurrent infections, family history and abdominal or joint pain since childhood. The tests used are :

II.1.9.1. EMMEL or sodium metabisulphite technique

*18+ This based on sickle cell transformation; it is only of orientation value and does not allow the different forms of sickle cell disease to be differentiated. Its aim is to identify sickle cell disease by depriving the red blood cell of oxygen.

II.1.9.2. Blood count :

It may reveal a constant but variable, regenerative anaemia often around 6 to 8g/dl Hb *6+.

II.1.9.3. DNA analysis of foetal fibroblasts: This is used for prenatal diagnosis *18+.

II.1.9.4. Dithionite-urea test or ITANO test:

This is a simple screening test based on the precipitation of HbS in a reversible reducing medium after the addition of *6+ Urea. These tests can guide the diagnosis, but only Hb electrophoresis can confirm the diagnosis by specifying the form of haemoglobinopathy.

II.1.9.5. Electrophoresis of Hb: [6]

It is performed at alkaline pH on a cellulose acetate support or at acid pH on an agar citrate gel. It confirms the diagnosis by demonstrating the presence of HbS at a very high level (90 to 97%); the absence of adult Hb A; and the presence of Hb F to a greater or lesser extent (particularly in infants).

II.1.9.6. Isoelectrofocussing test in neonates

This is a pH gradient polyacrylamide gel electrophoresis technique using high voltage. It allows better characterisation of Hb structural variants, highlighting subtle differences in isoelectric point. Abnormal haemoglobins can thus be detected even in newborns.

II.1.10. Clinical forms :

II.1.10.1. Homozygous form

This presents as a chronic haemolytic anaemia interspersed with attacks of acute anaemia and CVO, often complicated by severe bacterial infections. It is sometimes asymptomatic for up to 5 to 6 months because the red blood cells contain a high level of HbF, which prevents sickle cell formation. Hb electrophoresis shows 90-97% HbS and 3-10% HbF *10+.

II.1.10.2. Heterozygous form

Asymptomatic as a rule, without anaemia and with a normal life expectancy. Abdominal, osteoarticular or neurological CVO have been reported in association with infection, exertion or hypoxia. The noisy forms probably correspond to β thalasso sickle cell disease and not to true heterozygous sickle cell disease. The presence of acute haemolysis should prompt a search for another cause, such as G6PD deficiency. Hb electrophoresis reveals the presence of HbA and HbS, but at a level below 50% in the majority of cases *10+.

II.1.10.3. Associated shapes :

Associate another haemoglobinopathy haemoglobinosis S.

- Double heterozygous S/C: This is the most common haemoglobinosis after sickle cell anaemia and is characterised by the presence of two hemoglobinoses, S and C, in heterozygous form. It is particularly common in the black population of West Africa. The pathophysiological basis of double heterozygosity SC is the same as that of sickle cell disease SS: it is the sickling of red blood cells that causes the clinical manifestations [19].

Hb electrophoresis no HbA, HbS and HbC are equal (45-55%), HbF varies from 2-10%, i.e. slightly lower than in SS forms, and HbA2 is normal at 1-3% [10].

- Sickle-cell anaemia: These are common and must be subdivided according to the β+ or β° type of thalassaemia. There are two modes of expression of S/β+ thalassaemia, one severe where the HbA does not exceed 15% and the other fairly benign where the HbA is around 25%. The clinical expression is quite variable in its severity, which is generally comparable to that of homozygous S/β° thalassaemia *10+.

- Other types: [6]

These are hereditary persistence of foetal Hb; hemoglobinosis D Punjad; sickle cell disease S/O Arab and sickle cell disease A/S Antilles.

II. 1.11. Treatment :

II.1.11.1. Therapeutic management: [4]

The aim of this update is not to deal with the complete treatment of sickle cell disease. However, certain elements are fundamental to improving the disease's outcome.

➢ Treatment of CVO :

Pain treatment and protection of infarct tissues [6].

An early bone crisis can be treated at home with analgesics and hyperhydration. If treatment fails within 24 hours, the patient should be admitted to hospital. This does not apply to infants, who must be admitted to hospital immediately *4+.

In hospital, two therapeutic actions are carried out together: pain relief and hyperhydration.

➢ Painkillers: Pain is treated in stages, from level I analgesics to morphine, based on a very close assessment pain intensity using age-appropriate assessment scales [4].

➢ Hyperhydration: [20]

The theoretical basis for this practice is the cellular dehydration of sickle cell red blood cells linked to the Gardos effect and the increase in blood viscosity at steady state and its accentuation during CVO. The hyperhydration solution used is isotonic glucose serum (IGS) to which is added bicarbonate, the beneficial effects of which in sickle cell anaemia have not been demonstrated, is not used unless there are signs of acidosis.

For oral hyperhydration, coconut milk, which is much appreciated, is widely recommended, as are tap water, local fruit juices and other sweet drinks. In practice, in cases of severe CVO, intravenous infusion is the rule: 3l/m2/24hours, i.e. 150ml/kg/24hours. Oral hyperhydration, although less effective, may be prescribed, but mainly on an outpatient basis.

➢ Oxygen therapy: is indicated if necessary.

➢ Antibiotic therapy: discussed on a basis, targeted at pneumococcus or extended but it is not systematic. It can even be done in the absence of fever if a bacterial infection is suspected or diagnosed *20+.

➢ Transfusion: The aim is correct poorly tolerated anaemia and reduce the hbS level in order to prevent the consequences of sickle cell disease. This is either a simple transfusion or a *21+ exchange transfusion.

- Simple transfusion: This is indicated in the event of any clinically poorly tolerated drop in Hb levels (acute splenic sequestration; acute erythroblastopenia; acute thoracic syndrome; acute neurological accident; preparation for long-term surgery).

- Exchange transfusion: This is a transfusion carried out at the same time as bloodletting, in order to achieve isovolaemic exchange. It is carried out either occasionally or on a long-term basis (programmed exchange). ▪ One-off exchange: its indications are varied: Stroke, hyperalgesic CVO resistant to major analgesics, arterial thrombosis, failure of etilefrine in priapism, perioperative etc.

▪ Scheduled exchange: this is an absolute indication in cases previous stroke (ineffectiveness of hdroxyurea) in order to maintain hbS levels of< 30%, which are necessary to prevent recurrences. An exchange is performed every 4 to 6 weeks.

II.12.2 Preventive measures :

They are based on the prevention of CVO or haemolytic crises and infectious complications during follow-up of the sickle cell child *5+.
These preventive measures must be applied from childhood. However, sickle cell syndromes are still diagnosed late in Africa because there no systematic neonatal screening programme*19+.
These measures include :

► CVO prevention :

The aim is to avoid triggering factors, promote a regular, balanced diet, and recommend adequate water intake, particularly during feverish periods, during exercise and in hot climates *11+. Finally, any condition likely to cause hypoxia should be treated vigorously *4+.

► Preventing infection :

It is essential in tropical environments. It should concern SS patients as well as composite heterozygotes who are also subject to functional asplenia and the risk of serious infections *4, 5, 19, 20+.

▪ Oral penicillin is given systematically from the age of 3 months, with daily administration of oral penicillin in 2 or 3 doses, up to the age of 5, at doses ranging from 50,000 to 100,000 IU/kg/day.

▪ Vaccination with pneumococcal conjugate vaccine at 2, 3 and 4 months, with a booster at 16-18 months.

▪ All vaccines must be carried out regularly and renewed. These include the EPI and the vaccines particularly recommended for sickle cell patients, which are the vaccines against haemophilus influenzae b, pneumo 23 at the age of 2 with a booster every 3 years, and the A+C meningitis vaccination, which is highly recommended [4].

▪ Other anti-infectious prophylactic measures need to be taken, particularly against malaria and intestinal parasitosis.

Promote the use of insecticide-treated mosquito nets during the rainy season *5+.

As for the prevention of intestinal parasitosis, this is justified by the extreme frequency of these diseases among children in the African context. Systematic deworming with Albendazole is recommended for children aged 0-5 years.

▪ The prevention of post-transfusion viral infections is based on the rational use of transfusions, but above all on systematic screening blood donors for HIV infection and hepatitis C and B.

These measures should be combined with folic acid supplementation, which is particularly useful in Africa where the diet generally does not provide sufficient folates [5].

It must be prescribed continuously for life to compensate for the needs arising from the intense regenerative activity of the bone marrow *4+. We prescribe a dose of 5 to 10 mg/day for 15 days/month. However, is important to explain the benefits and procedures to parents to avoid abandoning the treatment when the disease is only slightly symptomatic. Iron supplementation at a dose of 3 to 5 mg/kg/day for two to three months in any child presenting with a fall in baseline Hb and reticulocyte count associated with microcytosis and hypochromia of recent onset *5+.

► Genetic counselling: its aim is to detect, inform and prevent. One of these means of action is prenatal diagnosis (PND), which allows couples at genetic risk (AS, A beta thalassaemia) to have a diagnosis made on the foetus at the start of pregnancy by analysis of the DNA of fibroblasts or on foetal blood collected. However, the disadvantage is that this diagnosis raises serious ethical and psychological issues [6].

► Monitoring: Monitoring of the sickle cell child should be regular and not overly restrictive. It consists of monitoring the basal state (blood count and reticulocytes), detecting complications and ensuring good prevention of these complications [4].

II.1.11.3 Basic treatment

Its aim is to reduce the frequency of CVO as much as possible and improve the quality of life of these patients. These are inducers of foetal haemoglobin synthesis:

Hydroxy urea (Hydréa):

This antineoplastic inhibits DNA synthesis and increases the concentration of HbF in red blood cells. It has been used for some years in sickle cell disease to reduce the number of *4+ sickle cell crises. It also reduces endothelial adhesion receptors, thereby reducing the frequency of *6+ CVOs. Numerous experimental studies suggest that, in addition to these effects, hydroxy urea may reduce the inflammatory phenomena that contribute vascular obstruction. It is indicated for patients with frequent painful attacks and for those with recurrent thoracic syndromes. Some authors also recommend it in cases of very severe anaemia and in many situations requiring transfusion programmes, which it replaces.

Recombinant human erythropoietin :

Used alone or in combination with hydroxy urea, it could be synergistic with the reactivity of HbF synthesis induced by the latter, and could therefore be indicated in sickle cell patients who are insufficiently protected from painful attacks by Hydrea. The dosage required is not yet known.

Butyrate and its derivatives :

They act directly on the promoter of the gamma gene responsible for the synthesis of the gamma chain of Hb F *6+.

Transmembrane ion transport modifiers :

They reduce erythrocyte dehydration by inhibiting the activity of membrane channels responsible for water loss. These are the calcium-dependent Gardos channel, inhibited by the administration of oral clotrimazole, and the channel responsible for KCL co-transport, which can be inhibited by magnesium. They are still at the clinical trial stage*6,13+.

Familial allogeneic marrow or cord blood transplants:

This is the only curative therapy for sickle cell disease. Its aim is to replace SS red blood cells with AA or AS red blood cells, thereby eliminating complications and possibly repairing existing lesions. It is only possible if there is a potential HLA-compatible donor in the patient's family who is heterozygous or free of the trait. The indications are recurrent thoracic syndromes, severe and recurrent CVO, stroke and recurrent priapism. The disadvantage is rejection in 10-15%, mortality around 10% and very high cost *6+.

Gene therapy :

This is a cutting-edge technique which involves acting directly on the genes responsible for the disease. In the case of sickle cell anaemia, the patient's bone marrow is taken, the cells are genetically modified with a therapeutic protein and reinjected into the patient, whose red blood cells will then function normally for good*7+.

II .2. DESCRIPTION OF THE PAINFUL SICKLE CELL CRISIS :

II.2.1. Pathophysiology :

The occurrence of CVOs can be explained by two phenomena:

II.2.1.1. Avascular necrosis of the bone marrow: [10]

It is due to infarctions caused by sickle red blood cells in the haematopoietic bone marrow and is responsible osteonecrosis manifested by painful bone crises such as the "foot-hand" syndrome, osteoarticular pain, abdominal pain due to avascular necrosis of the spine or a lower rib (painful projection into the abdomen).

II.2.1.2. Vaso-occlusion proper :

It results from obstruction of blood vessels by rigid, high-viscosity sickle red blood cells, leading to downstream infarction in the corresponding territory with tissue anoxia [10]. In fact, the red blood cell does not behave as a passive container for Hb, but has a whole series of functions which may contribute to pathophysiology. , it has been demonstrated that red blood cells highly heterogeneous, the most obvious heterogeneity being linked to their age. There is an abundant reticulocytic population which retains a number of characteristics which may paradoxically contribute to vaso-obstructive phenomena.

Vaso-obstruction can be modelled as a localised and multifactorial microvascular collapse which is sine qua non dependent on the presence of red blood cells with little or no deformability. Some studies have demonstrated the contribution of neutrophils to the risk of these accidents. The coagulation system the broad sense is moderately activated, but does not appear to play more than a secondary role in this very specific type of thrombosis *13+.

II.2.2. Semiology of CVO pain

The onset of intermittent, generally unpredictable and recurrent attacks of moderate or severe pain. There no explanation for the wide clinical variability. *3+. The first signs appear in the first few months of life, and more rarely after the age of 4-5 years. These are acute complications with a background of chronic haemolytic anaemia. They are irregular, generally unpredictable and may occur spontaneously or be provoked by any situation leading to hypoxaemia. It can occur in the body, most commonly in the spine, knee, ankle, elbow and femur, but several sites may in succession during the same attack*22+. Other symptoms include headaches, dental pain, priapism and foot-and-hand syndrome or dactylitis in infants*3+. The type is rapidly maximal, deep, gnawing or throbbing, sometimes oppressive, exacerbated by mobilisation with an average duration of two to three days *a few hours to one or two weeks+. Spontaneous resolution may be rapid or progressive over several days. Physical examination is usually normal, although there may be some local redness and slight swelling; muscle contractures and stiffness; pain on palpation and a slight rise in temperature *3,22+.

II.2.2.1. Abdominal pain: [8]

They occur in isolation or in association with osteoarticular crises, especially in children, and vary in intensity and topography. They may last 3 to 5 days and then gradually subside. Signs of paralytic ileus, vomiting and cessation of bowel movements and gas are highly suggestive. They are often accompanied by fever, distension and abdominal defence. emergency diagnosis is a delicate one, and other acute abdominal conditions must be discussed in detail. as in a child without sickle cell disease. The frequency and severity of pyelonephritis, which may be the cause of febrile abdominal pain, should be emphasised, as should the more rare occurrence of episodes of abdominal pain associated with cardiac liver in the case of advanced sickle cell cardiopathy. An abdominal pain syndrome may be associated with papillary necrosis, which is not uncommon in major sickle cell syndromes, but also in AS forms.

II.2.2.2. **Osteoarticular pain :**

Their mechanism is linked to ischaemia secondary to obliteration of the micro-circulation in the bone, peri-articular and soft tissue territories. Inflammation follows.

➢ Foot-hand syndrome or dactylitis: [15]

Specific to sickle-cell anaemia infants and sickle-cell anaemia, it is the most common and often revealing manifestation of the disease during first year of life.

It reflects CVO of the extremities, involving the small carpals, tarsals, metacarpals and metatarsals, and often the phalanges. Involvement is acute and transient. Dactylitis may sometimes regress without sequelae; it may be limited to one hand or one foot. The clinical picture is characterised by acute swelling of the dorsal surface of the corresponding soft tissue, which is very painful, total functional impotence and fever.

The course is usually favourable, with spontaneous regression in one to three weeks. However, superinfection is possible, resulting in acute dactylitis, which later becomes osteomyelitis of the hand or foot. The causative organism is almost always salmonella.

X-rays initially show only soft tissue oedema; around the tenth day, periosteal appositions and areas osteoporosis and condensation appear; scintigraphy is very effective.

➢ Osteoarticular pain children and adults:

Bone and joint damage in sickle cell disease is very common; it occurs early and is responsible for the most severe disabilities in adulthood. Painful attacks of the long bones are the most typical, as are peri-articular pains. They may be single or multiple, often preceded by discomfort or local pain a few hours earlier. A full-blown attack almost always leads to local impotence, and the often very violent pain prevents the child from moving spontaneously.

These clinical features may stimulate rheumatic fever or acute arthritis. The vertebrae are often affected and the chondrosternal regions may be affected, giving precordial or thoracic pain which stimulates pericarditis or pleuropneumonia. These attacks last approximately 3 to 4 days.

II.2.2.3. Chest pain: [23]

Acute pulmonary complications in sickle cell disease are frequent and are grouped together under the term acute chest syndrome or ACUTE CHEST SYNDROM. It is a major cause of death in patients with sickle cell disease. Clinically, it is defined by the combination of chest pain, dyspnoea and chest radiological signs. It constitutes a diagnostic and therapeutic emergency. It is likely that a number of less typical cases of acute chest syndrome are confused with acute lower respiratory infections, namely pneumonia and bronchopneumonia. The precise aetiology remains undetermined in more than half of cases. In addition to oxygen therapy, treatment requires hyperhydration, analgesia, exchange transfusion or, failing that, a simple transfusion.

II.2.2.4. Priapism :

Defined as a prolonged and often painful erection, it is a rare urological emergency in children *24+. Due to uni or bilateral thrombosis of the corpora cavernosa. This is one of the most severe forms of CVO and one of the major complications of sickle cell disease because of the pain and discomfort it causes and, above all, the sexual impotence it can lead to as a result of secondary fibrosis of the corpora cavernosa [11].

It is most often secondary to sickle cell anaemia and occurs mainly at night. Sexual intercourse and physiological nocturnal erections, which generate stasis in the corpora cavernosa, are thought to play a contributory role. Acute priapism (lasting more than 3 hours) requires urgent puncture and lavage of the corpora cavernosa to avoid permanent functional damage. It is almost always preceded by spontaneously resolving episodes of intermittent priapism*11+.

The efficacy of the alpha stimulant (etilefrin) in children with sickle cell disease in both intermittent priapism and acute priapism treated at an early stage has been demonstrated*24+.

Priapism often subsides within a few hours with hyperhydration. As with major CVO, prolonged or recurrent priapism is a broad indication for exchange transfusion *11+.

II. 3. PAIN MANAGEMENT ACCORDING TO WHO CRITERIA

II.3.1. PAIN ASSESSMENT :

- Self-assessment (25)

It concerns children aged 6 or over and was carried out using the EVA scale (visual analogue scale). This is a quick and easy method of self-assessment (by the child him/herself) from the age of 6: it is a 10 cm line marked by a ruler fitted with a cursor defined by two ends: on one side there is no pain and on the other maximum pain, the worst imaginable. During an attack, all degrees of pain are possible, from mild to extreme.

INTERPRETATION : 1-3: pain of mild intensity

4-5: moderate pain 6-10: severe pain

- . Hetero-evaluation: (26)

It concerns children under the age of 6, and is based on the use of behavioural measures. It was carried out using the Gustave Roussy DEGR scale (pain in children), which defines pain in terms of three parameters: psychomotor atony, analgesic positions and complaints.

	CONTRIBUTION				
PARAMETRES	0	1	2	3	4
1. ANTALGIC POSITIONAT REST	ABSENT	THE CHILD AVOIDS CERTAIN POSITIONS	HE AVOIDS CERTAIN NON-VISIBLE POSITIONS	HE CHOOSES A PAIN-RELIEVING POSITION	HE LOOKS FOR THE POSITION BUT CAN'T FIND IT
2.MISSING D'EXPRESSIVITE	THE LIVELY, DYNAMIC CHILD	HE LOOKS DARK	AT LEAST ONE OF THE SIGNS : FEATURE FROM FACE LITTLE EXPRESSIVE ;REGARD MORNE	ALL THE SIGNS OF 2 TOGETHER	FUGE FACE AS IF ENLARGED
3. SPONTANEOUS PROTECTION OF ZONES DOULOUREUSES	IL DOES PROTECT ITSELF	HE AVOIDS VIOLENT CLASHES	HE PROTECTS HIS BODY	IT LIMITS ALL TOUCHING	ALL THE CARE REQUIRED TO PROTECT
4. SOMATIC COMPLAINTS SEU	NOT FROM COMPLAINTS	COMPLAINT WITHOUT EMOTIONAL EXPRESSION	EXPRESSIVE FACIAL EXPRESSION NT LA PLAI NTE	HE ATTIRE ATTENTION TO SAY THAT IT HURTS	GEMINATION ACCOMPANYING THE PAIN
5.DESINTERET FOR THE WORLD EXTERNAL	HE IS INTERESTED IN THE ENVIRONMENT WITH ENERGY	HE IS INTERESTED IN THE ENVIRONMENT ENT	HE'S BORED	UNABLE TO PLAY	HE IS INDIFFERENT

INTERPRETATION: Moderate pain if DEGR$\leq$ to 16 Intense pain if DEGR> to 16.

II.3.2. **Treatment of painful crisis: (26)**

➤ Analgesics :

Pain is treated in stages using analgesics based on the WHO classification.

Mild pain: Level I analgesics with or without oral NSAIDs as an outpatient.

▪ Paracetamol: 10-15mg/kg/every 4 to 6 hours.

▪ Niflumic acid: 40 mg/kg/day orally, as a gel or intrarectally (from 10 kg).
▪ Ibuprofen: 10 mg/kg/6 to 8 hours; suppository and drinkable suspension for infants aged 6 months and over, and tablets for older children.

▪ ASPIRIN: 25 to 50 mg/kg every 6 .

▪ Ketoprofen (Profenid*): ½ tablet to 1 tablet every 8 .

Moderate pain of moderate intensity: Level I and/or II analgesics, with or without NSAIDs. Day hospital or inpatient treatment: parenteral route followed by oral route.

▪ Paracetamol injection (perfalgan*):15mg/kg every 6 hours by slow infusion over 15 minutes.

▪ Ketoprofen injection (Profenid*): 25 to 75 mg/kg or 1 to 2 ampoules on receipt diluted in 100 ml of 5% glucose, then 1 ampoule every 8 hours intramuscularly.

▪ Temgesic injectable 0.3 mg/ml: 1 ampoule every 12 hours by slow intravenous or intramuscular injection; or sublingual 0.2 mg/ml every 8 hours at a dose of 15 to 25μg/kg.

Intense pain: pure strong agonist opioids with no ceiling dosage These are necessary for all severe pain. These drugs are simple to administer and effectively relieve pain in the majority of children. The strong opioid of choice on the WHO model list of essential medicines is morphine; its substitutes are hydromorphone, methadone and fentanyl. Pethidine is not recommended for prolonged use because of the accumulation of its toxic metabolite.

ORAL MORPHINE

Immediate-release morphine :

▪ Morphine hydrochloride: in most children the recommended initial dose is 0.15-0.3 mg/kg every 4 hours, adjusted individually until pain is sedated.

▪ Morphine sulphate: Actiskenan* - Sustained-release morphine

▪ Skenan*, tablet 1 dose/12 hours.

▪ Kapanol, at a dose of 0.6 mg/kg every 8 hours or 0.9 mg/kg every 12 hours. Oral preparations of morphine sulphate and hydrochloride are available.

Aqueous solutions are bitter, so children prefer the medicine mixed with a flavoured syrup.

™ Morphine injection :

Its routes of administration are: subcutaneous; intravenous; epidural at a dose of 0.15-0.3 mg/kg/4 hours.

™ Contraindications to morphine :

▪ Respiratory failure ;

▪ Occlusive syndrome ;

▪ Diagnostic uncertainty regarding the abdomen.

™Side effects of oral morphine :

When prescribed as recommended, morphine does not cause respiratory depression, occlusion, prolonged sedation, mental disorders or drug dependence. Patients or their parents should be informed of the possibility of the four most common side effects: constipation, vomiting, drowsiness and nausea. Other side effects are possible but rare: hallucinations; confusion; dysphonia; dizziness; nightmares; waking with a start; myoclonus; urinary retention; sweating; pruritus. Constipation is a constant undesirable effect, and morphine prescriptions must be accompanied by a prescription for a laxative, as is codeine.

➢ General measures

- Hyperhydration: 150 ml/kg/day. The parenteral route was used for moderate to severe seizures and the oral route for mild seizures.
- Rest, immobilisation of painful limbs.
- Oxygenation: if hypoxia associated.
- Antibiotics: not useful for pain, but indicated if there is the slightest doubt.
- Transfusion if necessary, but the impact on pain itself has never been assessed.

MATERIALS AND METHODS

II.1. MATERIAL

A. HUMAN RESOURCES

II.1.1. FRAMEWORK OF THE STUDY :

Our study was carried out in the paediatric ward of the Centre de Médecine Mixte et d'Anémie SS. This centre is located in the commune of Kalamu, Funa district, Kinshasa/DRC.

II.1.2. PERIOD OF STUDY :

Our study covered the period from 1st January to 31 December 2018.

II.1.3. STUDY POPULATION :

Our study population consisted of children with sickle cell disease aged between 6 months and 17 years.

II.1.4. INCLUSION AND NON-INCLUSION

III.4.1. INCLUSION :

Individuals meeting the following criteria were included in our study:

- Children aged 6 months to 17 years, regardless of gender;
- Known or confirmed sickle cell disease;
- Be admitted to the paediatric ward with a history of vaso-occlusive crises during the period in question.

III.3.2. NON-INCLUSION CRITERIA :

Patients with incomplete records were excluded.

B. NON-HUMAN MATERIALS

To carry out our work, we mainly used :

- Paediatric department register

➢ Patient medical records

➢ Data collection sheets

➢ Laptop computer

II.2. METHODS :

II.2.1. TYPE OF STUDY :

This is a documentary and retrospective study.

II.2.2. SAMPLE SIZE :

Our sample size consisted of all children who met the inclusion criteria.

II.2.3. Sampling technique :

We proceeded by an exhaustive sampling of cases.

III.2.4. Parameters of interest

CATEGORIES	PARAMETERS
SOCIO-DEMOGRAPHIC	Breakdown of patients by: age group; sex; school performance; sibling rank
CLINICS	Distribution of patients according to sickle cell in the family;time of onset of the 1st CVO;notion of syndrome hands-feet;monthly frequency of painful attacks, factors triggering the attack;site of pain;weight;intensity of pain
PARACLINIQUES	Breakdown of patients by: haemoglobin electrophoresis; other tests performed (GE, Rx, etc.); associated pathologies
TREATMENT	Distribution of patients according to: analgesic level; associated or adjuvant treatment; length of hospital stay,

III.2.5. OPERATIONAL DEFINITIONS :

a. Frequency: a characteristic that occurs at more or less frequent intervals.

b. Socio-demographic factor: this is a population segmentation criterion based on variables such as age, gender, housing, etc.

c. Siblings: all brothers and sisters in the same family

d. Analgesics or painkillers: these are drugs designed to reduce pain.

e. Pain: an physical sensation, emotion or feeling; generally speaking, we talk about pain when the patient says it hurts.

f. Crisis: sudden onset of an illness or sudden worsening of a chronic condition.

III.2.6. DATA PROCESSING :

The data collected was entered and analysed on the computer using Microsoft Office Excel 2013. Statistical analyses carried out using IBM IPSS software (the statistical package for the social sciences). The results were presented in the form of scientific tables.

III.2.7. ETHICAL CONSIDERATIONS :

Our work was carried out in strict compliance with ethical principles. Only the principal investigator and the supervisor managed the data collected, and they did so confidentially and anonymously.

RESULTS

II.3. FREQUENCY

In our work we enrolled for the period from January to December 2018, 220 children with sickle cell disease admitted with a vaso-occlusive crisis, out of a total of 1520 admissions; a frequency of 14.5%.

II.4. SOCIO-DEMOGRAPHIC CHARACTERISTICS

The tables I, II, III and IV give the different socio-demographic characteristics of patients.

Table I. Breakdown of patients by age group

Age groups (years)	Workforce	Percentage
'1	0	0
1-5	53	24,1
6-10	88	40
11-15	71	32,3
'15	8	3,64
TOTAL	220	100

The table shows that the 6 to 10 year age group was the most represented, with 40% of patients, and no patient was less than one year old. The average age of patients was 9 years. The extremes were 1 year and 17 years.

Table II: Breakdown of patients by sex

SEX	WORKFORCE	PERCENTAGE
MALE	123	55,91
WOMEN	97	44,09
TOTAL	220	100

The table shows that 55.91% of the patients were male. The sex ratio was 1.23.

Table III below shows the distribution of patients according to their school performance. It should be noted that of the 220 patients, only 96 had a school leaving certificate.

Table III: Distribution of patients according to school performance

SCHOOL LEVEL	WORKFORCE	PERCENTAGE
EDUCATIONAL DELAY	53	55,21
NO EDUCATIONAL DELAY	43	44,79
TOTAL	96	100

This table shows that 64 patients did not reach school age and 60 did. but had not studied. The majority of patients (55.21%) were behind at school.

Table IV: Breakdown of patients by sibling rank

Sibling rank	Workforce	Percentage
1e	58	26,4
2e	95	43,2
3e	39	17,73
'3	28	12,73
TOTAL	220	100

Patients with the ^{2nd} most siblings predominate (43.2%)

II.5. BACKGROUND

Table V: Distribution of patients according to the number of sickle cell patients in the family

Sickle cell disease in the family	Workforce	Percentage(%)
1	184	83,63
2	34	15,5
3	2	0,91
TOTAL	220	100

The vast majority (83.63%) of our patients were the only sickle cell patients in their siblings.

Table VI: Distribution of patients according to the time of onset of the 1st vaso-occlusive attack

Age of first attack (years)	Workforce	Percentage
'1	40	18,2
1-2	168	76,4
≥3	8	3,64
7	1	0,45
NOT specified	3	1,36
TOTAL	220	100

This table shows that in the majority of cases, the 1st vaso-occlusive crisis was between the ages of 1-2 years.

Table VII: Distribution of patients according to the notion of hand-foot syndrome

Hand foot syndrome	Workforce	Percentage
No	184	83,64
Yes	36	16,36
TOTAL	220	100

Hand-foot syndrome did not occur in 83.64% of patients.

Table VIII: Breakdown of patients by monthly frequency of attacks painful

Monthly frequency of attacks	Workforce	Percentage
1	78	35,46
2	129	58,64
3	13	5,91
TOTAL	220	100

Patients experiencing 2 attacks a month are the most represented, with 58.64%.

II.6. CLINICAL DATA :

Table IX: Breakdown of patients according to factors triggering the crisis

Triggering factor	Workforce	Percentage
Intense effort	75	34,1
Fever	97	44,1
Cold	48	21,8
TOTAL	220	100

Fever is the most common, at 44.1%.

Table X: Breakdown of patients by site of pain

Site of pain	Workforce	Percentage(%)
Thoracic	5	2,3
Abdominal	42	19,1
OSTEOARTICULAR	150	68,2
ABDO AND THORACIC	1	0,45
ABDO AND OSTEOARTICULAR	22	10
TOTAL	220	100

Osteoarticular pain accounted for 68.2%

Table XI: Breakdown of patients by weight

Weight	Workforce	Percentage
Normal weight	77	35
UNDERWEIGHT	143	65
TOTAL	220	100

The majority of patients (65%) had a delay in their weight and height.

Table XII: Distribution of patients according pain intensity

INTENSITY OF PAIN	WORKFORCE	PERCENTAGE
1-3	34	32,7
4-5	25	24,04
6-10	45	43,3
TOTAL	104	100

There were 116 patients whose pain was not assessed. In our sample, the majority of painful attacks were severe (43.3%).

Table XIII: Distribution of patients according to the time taken to sedate with analgesics

SEDATION TIME to analgesics (H)	WORKFORCE	PERCENTAGE
2	155	70,5
3	30	13,6
24	35	15,9
TOTAL	220	100

This table shows that the effectiveness of analgesic was assessed at 2th hour in 70% of cases, with an average of 13 hours.

Table XIV: Breakdown of patients by time to seizure sedation

SEIZURE SEDATION TIME	WORKFORCE	PERCENTAGE
≤6	40	18,2
6 and ≤12	70	31,8
'12	110	50
TOTAL	220	100

50% of our patients' pain subsided within more than 12 hours, with an average of 9 hours.

Table XV: Distribution of patients according age at ^{1st} attack and monthly frequency of attacks

age frequency	1	2	3
6 MONTHS	11	27	2
12 MONTHS	34	44	4
24 MONTHS	30	51	5
36 MONTHS	2	4	2
84 MONTHS	1	0	0
NO	0	3	0

The majority of patients, whether or not the age of first attack is known, have 2 painful attacks per month, with a predominance in those aged 24 months.

Table XVI: Breakdown of patients by pain trigger and site

Seat Factor	Thoracic	Abdominal	Osteoarticular	Abdo and thoracic	Abdo and osteoarticular
Intense effort	0	8	58	0	9
Fever	3	22	63	1	8
Cold	2	12	29	0	5

Whatever the triggering factor, the predominant site of pain is osteoarticular.

Table XVII: Breakdown of patients by age group and triggering factors

Factor age	INTENSE EFFORT	FEVER	COLD
6-60 MONTHS	10	24	19
72-120 MONTHS	31	43	14
132-204 MONTHS	34	30	15

Fever is the predominant trigger for pain in the 6-60 and 72-120 month age groups, while intense effort is the main trigger for pain in the 132-204 month age group.

Table XVIII: Breakdown of patients by monthly frequency of attacks and weight

Weight Frequency	Normal weight	Delayed growth and weight
1	27	51
2	45	84
3	5	8

Delayed growth and weight are predominant in all monthly frequencies of painful attacks.

Table XIX: Breakdown by monthly frequency of crises and school level

SCHOLARSHIP FREQUENCY OF CRISES	Normal schooling	School delay
1	14	22
2	27	27
3	2	4

Patients with normal schooling or a delay in schooling have proportionately more than 2 painful attacks per month.

II.7. PARACLINICAL DATA

Table XX: Distribution of patients according haemoglobin electrophoresis

Electrophoresis HB	Workforce	Percentage
SS	188	85,45
AS	32	14 ,55
TOTAL	220	100

Homozygotes predominate with 85.45%.

Table XXI: Distribution of patients according to haemoglobin admission

Hb level	Workforce	Percentage
5	1	0,45
6	15	6,82
7	50	22,73
8	123	55,91
9	31	14,1
TOTAL	220	100

This table shows that in the majority of cases, the haemoglobin admission was 8g/dl at 55.91%.

Table XXII: Breakdown of patients by associated pathologies

Associated pathology	Workforce	Percentage
ENT INF.	3	3
INTESTINAL PARASITOSIS	24	24
MALARIA	64	64
PNEUMONIA	5	5
SEPSIS	4	4
TOTAL	100	100

120 patients had no associated pathologies. Malaria predominated (64%).

II.8. TREATMENT

Table XXIII: Distribution of patients according to analgesic level

Analgesic level	Workforce	Percentage
Level I	115	52,27
Stage II	105	47,73
TOTAL	220	100

The most commonly used analgesic level was level I with 52.27%.

Table XXIV: Breakdown of patients by use of anti-inflammatory drugs

Anti-inflammatory	Workforce	Percentage
YES	47	21,36%
NO	173	78,64
TOTAL	220	100

This table shows that in most cases, anti-inflammatory drugs were not used (78.64%).

Table XXV: Distribution of patients according to use alkaline hyperhydration

Alkaline hyperhydration	Workforce	Percentage
YES	69	31,36
NO	151	68,64
TOTAL	220	100

This table shows that alkaline hyperhydration was not used in most cases (68.64%).

Table XXVI: Breakdown of patients according to use of antispasmodics

Anti spasmodic	Workforce	Percentage
YES	47	21,36
NO	173	78,64
TOTAL	220	100

This table shows that in most cases, antispasmodics were not used (78.64%).

II.9. EVOLUTION

Table XXVII: Breakdown of patients by length of hospital stay

Length of hospital stay	Workforce	Percentage
2	4	1,82
3	32	14,55
4	40	18,2
5	83	37,7
6	16	7,3
7	20	9,1
8	3	1,36
9	2	0,91
11	1	0,45
14	4	1,82
21	4	1,82
30	6	2,73
60	3	1,36
74	1	0,45
90	1	0,45
TOTAL	220	100

This table shows that the predominant length hospitalisation was 5 days (37.7%), with an average length of hospitalisation of 22±93 days.

Table XXVIII: Distribution of patients according to monthly frequency of attacks and analgesic level

Bearing Frequency of attacks	Level I	Stage II
1	45	33
2	66	63
3	4	9

Despite the predominance of 2 attacks per month, the most commonly used analgesic level is level I.

Table XXIX: Distribution of patients according to pain intensity and analgesic level

Bearing Intensity of pain	Level I	Stage II
1-3(light)	27	7
4-5(moderate)	6	19
6-10(intense)	18	27
No	64	52

116 patients did not have their pain assessed. For mild intensity, the most used is Level I, but for moderate and intense intensity the most commonly used level is Level II.

Table XXX: Distribution of patients according to haemoglobin electrophoresis and monthly frequency of attacks

FREQUENCY ELECT. HB	1	2	3
SS	65	113	10
AS	13	16	3

These patients have more than 2 painful attacks per month, but the most at risk are homozygotes.

Table XXXI: Distribution of patients according outcome

Evolution	Workforce	Percentage
Good	125	56,82
Wrong	95	43,18
TOTAL	220	100

This table shows that most patients had a good outcome (56.82%).

Table XXXII: Distribution of patients according to the intensity of the crisis and the length of hospitalisation

DURATION INTEN.	2	3	4	5	6	≥7
1-3	1	5	6	13	4	5
4-5	3	2	4	12	1	3
6-10	12	8	1	20	1	3

This table shows that whatever intensity of the pain, the predominant day of hospitalisation is 5 days.

Table XXXIII: Breakdown of patients by length of hospital stay and associated pathologies

P.ASSOCIATES DURATION	ENT INF.	INTESTINAL PARASITOSIS	MALARIA	PNEUMONIA	SEPSIS
2	1	1	2	0	0
3	8	7	10	7	0
4	10	13	15	1	1
5	12	20	41	7	3
6	2	3	9	2	0
≥7	11	10	25	3	1

This table shows that whatever the length of hospitalisation, the most predominant associated disease is malaria.

COMMENTS AND DISCUSSIONS

In order to study the effectiveness of the WHO method of pain treatment by analgesic steps in sickle cell pain crises, we conducted a study in the paediatric department of the SS mixed medicine and anaemia centre on the management of sickle cell pain crises over a period from June to December 2019. In our study we included 220 patients. We chose age group 6 months to 17 years because it corresponded on the one hand to the population most affected by the painful sickle cell crisis and on the other hand because it was the paediatric age group which predominated during consultations during the above-mentioned period. In our sample, the average age of patients was 5 years, with extremes of 6 months and 17 years. The 72-120 month age group was the most affected with 40%, followed by the 132-204 month age group with 35.9%. In other studies, such as those by Thuilliez et al in 1987 (33) and C.O. Eloundou (31), 72 to 180 month age group was found to be predominant (63.33%). The same is true of Tall et al (34) and De Montalembert (35). Sickle cell pain attacks mainly affect children of school age; it cannot be ruled out that it may occur before this age. Our sample was dominated by males, who accounted for 55.91% of cases, followed by 44.09% of females, giving a sex ratio of 1.23 in favour of males. Rates comparable to ours were previously observed by D. Diallo (32) in 2004, i.e. 54.5%.Pichard et al. (36) in Mali found a clear male predominance with 70%.On the other hand, C.O.Eloundou(31) in 2002 found a female predominance in his study, i.e. 58.3%.The recent study by L.Dioné(37) found that the male sex was as well represented as the female sex, with 50% each. In our study, educational delay was observed in 55.21% of cases. Thuilliz et al (33) found a result close to ours (34%). In the study by C.O.Eloundou (31), 61% of cases were found to be behind school. This difference can probably be explained by the significant number (29.1%) of children who had not reached school age and 27.3% of those who had reached school age but were not studying in our study. The staturo-weight retardation usually encountered in sickle cell patients was also present in our study, with a predominance of 65%. C.O.Eloundou (31) found a result close to ours (30%), could be explained by the fact that underweight increases with age.In our study, the majority of sickle cell patients were homozygotes with a predominance of 85.5%, as in the studies by C.O.Eloundou(31) and in Gabon by Thuilliez et al. (33).Homozygotes are more likely to have attacks than heterozygotes. In our study 83.6% of the children were the only sickle cell patients in their siblings. C.OEloundou(31) found a similar result with 65% of cases. D. Diallo in his study found similar results with 69%(32).the age of the first painful attack was in the majority of cases around 2 years (39.1%).this result is contrary to that of C.O.Eloundou(31) who found a predominance around 6 months (38.2%) as is usual in this pathology. In our study we found a predominance of children having 2 seizures per month (58.64%); the Gabonese study by C.O. Eloundou(31) found predominance of children having one seizure per month. This diversity in frequency can be explained in part by the quality of care provided to these patients during the inter-critical period and also by genetic factors (30; 38).The majority of painful seizures triggered by fever (44.1%), favoured in our context by the endemic malaria (64%). The study by C.O.Eloundou(31) found similar results. On admission, the majority of seizures were severe (43.3%), followed by moderate seizures (24.04%), but 52.73% of the sample did not have their pain assessed. The predominant length hospitalisation was 5 days, i.e. 37.7 It is close to that of C.O.Eloundou(31) who found 3 days.68.2The C.OEloundou study(31) found similar results with 81.6% of attacks relieved by stage I analgesics; 18.3% required a switch to stage II analgesics.Pain sedation occurred after an average of 2 hours. Sangaré et al in Côte d'Ivoire *39+ in a therapeutic trial based on Buprenorphine (level II analgesic) obtained a sedation time of 2 days in 84% of patients, while Bègue and Castello-Hebreteau in France *40+ reported a treatment time of 4 to 5 days. Gbadoe et al *20+, like us, used stage I and II analgesics with good results. In Western countries, on the other hand, this WHO protocol very often mentions its tier III, with easier access to morphines if necessary.

CONCLUSION AND RECOMMENDATIONS

VI.a. CONCLUSION :

At the end of our study on the management of painful sickle cell crises in the paediatric department of SS mixed medicine and anaemia centre, we found that :
-Children aged between 72 and 120 months were the most affected (40%).
-Severe seizures on admission were the most common (43.3%), followed by moderate seizures (24.04%).
The majority of attacks were controlled with stage I analgesics (52.27%), not often associated with alkaline hyperhydration and non-steroidal anti-inflammatory drugs, with recourse to stage II analgesics in 47.73%.
-The assessment scales helped to systematise pain intensity, which seemed to have an influence on seizure sedation.
This analysis enabled us to demonstrate the effectiveness of this pain treatment method proposed by the WHO for painful sickle cell crises. It is generally known that in the absence of treatmentpainful sickle cell crises can last from a few hours to a few weeks.

VI.b. RECOMMENDATIONS

In view of the results obtained, we recommend : The health authorities to :
Provide hospitals with tier I analgesics and non-steroidal anti-inflammatory drugs as essential medicines;
-Initiate specialist training on sickle cell anaemia and retraining of community providers;
-Support the various associations involved in the fight against sickle cell disease and its complications
To the doctors of :
-Treat sickle cell disease as a public health problem requiring early and appropriate care;
-Familiarising nursing staff and patients with pain assessment scales and the use of hydroxy urea (hydrea) in our sanitary facilities;
-Using information, education and communication programmes, promote correct home analgesia, which has a real impact on the incidence of hospitalisation for these patients;

-Teach parents to recognise the triggers and warning signs.

To families:
-Ensure regular monitoring of children in order to apply preventive measures against the occurrence of seizures;
-Avoiding factors that encourage and trigger attacks;
Seek rapid medical attention in the event of an unbearable attack that is resistant to self-medication.

REFERENCES

1. N.Aloui*, N Nessib**, H.Darghouth*, I.Baccouche*, M.Sayed*, I.Bellagha*, F.Ben Chehida*, M.Ben Ghachem**, A.Hammou*. Contribution of MRI in febrile bone pain. Comparative study between vaso-occlusive crises in sickle cell disease and acute osteomyelitisë. WWW.biam2.org/biam.
2. M.Mbensa and A. Bolamba. Morbidity in major sickle cell disease in the urban environment of Kinshasa, DRC. Méd. d'Afrique noire: 1981,28(5).
3. E.Fournier-Charrière, J.P.Dommergues. Pain during sickle cell crisis in children: semiology, evaluation and treatment methods.
major painkillers. Ann. Pédiatre (Paris), 1995, 42, no 2, 105-114.
4. P. Begue & B.Castello-Herbreteau. Sickle cell disease in children and adolescents. Prise en charge en 2001 Bull Soc Pathol. Exot, 2001 94, 2 ; 85-89.
5. I.Diagne, N.D.R.Diagne-Gueye, H.Signate-Sy, B.Camara, PH.Lopez-Sall, A.Diack- M'baye, M.Sarr, M.Ba, H.D.Sow, N.Kuakuvi.
Management of sickle cell disease in children in Africa: experience of the cohort at the Albert Royer Children's Hospital in Dakar. Med .Trop 2003; 63: 513-520.
6. C. O. Eloundou. Management of painful sickle cell crisis according to WHO criteria. A study in a paediatric hospital in Libreville. Thèse méd. Bamako: 02-M- 32.
7. By Wal Fadjiri (Dakar) 28 January 2004 published on ufctogo.com 1 February 2004. Treatment of sickle-cell anaemia: Gene therapy to cure sickle-cell anaemia. http://www.ufctogo.com/article.php3?id article=263
8. M. Sangaré. Survey of health centre providers on the management of sickle cell disease in children in Bamako. Thèse méd. Bamako: 05-M-15.
9. D. Diallo. Suivi des enfants drépanocytaires de 0-15 ans dans le service de pédiatrie du CHU GT. Thèse méd. Bamako: 04 -M - 16.

10. C. Soumano. Knowledge and practical attitudes of mothers regarding care of sickle cell children in Bamako households. Thèse méd. Bamako: 05-M-16.
11. P. Beauvais. Drépanocytose expansion scientifique française 1981,98.616-15- BEA

12. French association for the screening and prevention of childhood disabilities. How to bring up a child with sickle cell disease. WWW.afdphe.ass.fr Edition May 2001.

13. F. Galacteros. Pathophysiological basis of sickle cell disease, management and current treatment. Bull Soc Pathol. Exot, 2001, 94, 2, 77-79.
14. I. Soares. Diagne, G.M.M, A**. Gueye, Diagne Gueye.ND.R.*, Fall.*,

B*.Camara, S*.Diouf, M*. Fall. Infections in Senegalese children and dolescents with sickle cell disease: epidemiological aspects. Dakar Médical, 2000, 45, 1,55-58.

15. Meddeb. Nihel*, Gandoura Najoua, Gandoura .Moncef ,Sellami.S. Manifestations ostéo- articulaires de la drépanocytose. La Tunisie médicale -vol : 81-No 07,2003 ; 441-447.

16. P.Acar*, C.Maunoury**, M de Montalembert*** and Y.Dulac*. Myocardial perfusion abnormalities in childhood sickle cell disease: a myocardial tomoscintigraphy study. Archives des maladies du cœur et des vaisseaux, tome 96, no 5, May 2003.

17. A. Tchango Kwethen. Renal manifestations associated with the sickle cell gene in the nephrology and haemodialysis department of the Hôpital du Point G in Bamako, Mali. Thesis med. Bamako: 2004-M-104.

18. Y. L. Diallo. Les complications ostéo-articulaires chez les drépanocytaires au Mali à propos de 31 cas. Thesis med. Bamako: 2001-M-50.

19. P.Aubry, E.TouzeJ. Double heterozygosity SC with osteonecrosis: a clinical case in tropical medicine. La Duraulie ed. 1990, pp.184-185.

20. A.D.Gdadoe*, N.Kampatibe**, B.Bakonde*, J.K.Assimadi*, K.Kessie. Therapeutic attitudes to sickle cell disease in the critical and inter-critical phases in Togo. Méd. d'Afrique Noire: 1998,45 (3).

21. M.C.Rahimy. Problems posed by transfusion children with sickle cell disease in Africa. Archives de pédiatrie 12 (2005) 802-804.

22. Pain in sickle cell disease. Page printed on http://WWW.ledamed.org.

23. Ammar Jamel-Ghrairi Hedia-El Mekki FathiA-Aissa Imen-Hamzaoui Agnès. Acute chest syndromes in sickle cell disease: surprising etiologies. A propos de trois cas avec revue de la littérature. Tunisie médicale- vol : 81-No05, 2003 ; 345-350.

24. H.Sibai*, A.Sakoute, M.Yaakoubi, M.Fehri. Priapism and pulmonary infection in children. Annales d'urologie 37 (2003) 143-145

25. MDe Montalembert. Emergencies children with sickle cell anaemia Réan. Intensive care. Méd. Urg. , 1994,10 (2) ; 81-87

26. AWA DEMBELE. Prise en charge de la crise douloureuse drépanocytaire selon les critères de l'OMS ; thèse de médecine 2008 ; 45-60

27. REGIONAL BLOOD TRANSFUSION CENTRE. Physiology of red blood cells and pathophysiology of anaemia; 2004: 62-83

28. Piel FB,Patil AP,Howes RE et al,Global epidemiology of sickle haemoglobin in neonates,Lancet.2013;381 (9861):142-5.PubMed/Google Scholar

29. ABDALA K.A.,MABIALA BABELA J.R.,SHINDANO M.E. Epidemiological, clinical and therapeutic aspects of sickle cell disease children at the Kindu general referral hospital, Rev.Afr.Méd et S.P/No 1-Vol. 2 June 2018.

30. E.Fournier-Charrière, J.P.Dommergues. Pain during sickle cell crisis children, semiology, evaluation and treatment methods: the role of major analgesics. Ann. Pédiatre (Paris), 1995, 42, no 2, 105-114.

31. C. O. Eloundou. Management of painful sickle cell crisis according to WHO criteria. A study in a paediatric hospital in Libreville. Thèse méd. Bamako: 02-M-32

32. D. Diallo. Suivi des enfants drépanocytaires de 0-15 ans dans le service de pédiatrie du CHU GT. Thèse méd. Bamako: 04 -M - 16.

33. V.Thuilliez, V.Ditsambou, JR.Mba, Mba. Meyo. S, J.Kitengue. Current aspects of sickle cell disease in children in Gabon.
Arch. Pédiatre 1996; 3 :668-74.

34. F.Talla , P.Agranat, O.Traoré , B.Nacro , A.Traoré. Sickle cell disease in paediatric patients in Burkina Faso. Drépanocytose et santé publique 1990 :165-74

35. M. De Montalembert, M.Guilloud. Bataille, J. Feingolde, R. Girot. Epidemiological and clinical study of sickle cell disease in France, French Guyana and Algeria. Eur. J. Haematol; 1993; 51:136-40

36. E.Pichar, B.Duflo, S.Coulibaly, B.Mariko, J.L.Mosempes, H.A.Traoré, A.D.Diallo. Evaluation of the efficacy of treatments during painful osteoarticular crises in sickle cell disease: the example of pentoxifylline. Bull .Soc.Path.Ex, 1987, 80 :834-40.

37. L .Dioné Les activités de l'unité fonctionnelle de prise en charge et de suivi des enfants drépanocytaires : Bilan d'une année au service de pédiatrie du CHU-GT. Thesis; Méd. 2007

38. A.Moussavoua*, Y.Vierina, C.Eloundou-Orima, M.Keitab. Pain management according to World Health Organisation criteria. Archives de pédiatrie 11 (2004) 1041-1045.

39. A.Sangaré, K.G.Koffio, L.Sanogo, A.H.Touré, A.Allangba, A.Tolo, F.H.Coulibaly, N'Dhatz, J.P.Elenga. Therapeutic trial of Buprenorphine (Temgesic) in the treatment of painful sickle cell crises. Méd. Afr. Noire 1998,45(2) :138-43

40. P. Begue & B.Castello-Herbreteau. Sickle cell disease in children and adolescents. Prise en charge en 2001 Bull Soc Pathol. Exot, 2001 94, 2 ; 85-89.

APPENDICES

LETTER OF ENQUIRY

I. PATIENT IDENTIFICATION

Q1 Name ; Post name :
Q2 Age :
Q3 Sex :
Q4 Address :
Q5 Sibling rank :
Q6 Level of education :
Q7 Number sickle cell children in the family: Q8 Haemoglobin electrophoresis :
Q9 Blood grouping :
Q10 Age of first attack :
Q11 Annual frequency of attacks :
Q12 Hand foot syndrome :

II. PHYSICAL EXAMINATION ON ENTRY

Q13 Weight :
Q14 Size :
Q15 Brachial perimeter :
Q16 Existence a staturo-ponderal delay yes or no Q17 Existence of an educational delay yes or no

III. ANALYSIS AND ASSESSMENT OF THE PAIN CRISIS

Q18 Pain assessed yes or no Q19 Intensity :
Q20 Location of pain :
Q21 Accompanying signs of pain: Q22 Factors triggering the attack :
1. physical effort 2.cold 3. fever 4.other: Q23 Associated pathologies :

IV. TREATMENT OF THE CRISIS

Q24 Treatment admission :Analgesic :
Antispasmodic: Alkaline hyperhydration: Anti-inflammatory:
Q25 Use other painkillers :
Q26 Adjuvant treatment :
Q27 Other treatments :

V. RESULT

Q28 Length hospitalisation for vaso-occlusive crisis

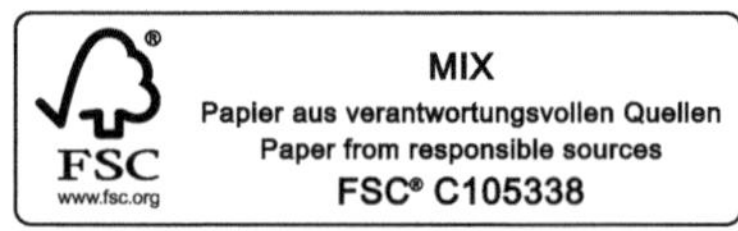

Printed by Books on Demand GmbH, Norderstedt / Germany